The Yoniverse:
Vaginal Detox Guide

YummyYoniPearls.net

What are Yummy Yoni Pearls?

Yummy Yoni Pearls are cloth-covered balls containing herbs, such as motherwort, osthol, angelica, borneol, and rhizome. The combination of herbs detoxes your womb and resets your natural balance, increasing elasticity, regulating the menstrual cycle, killing parasites and bacteria, improving fertility, reducing discharge, and removing toxins.

This guide is dedicated to the many goddesses who have trusted us with their womb detox journeys and have shared their journeys with others.

Thank you,

Jared & Mesi James

Table of Contents

Why should I detox my vagina?

Western medical professionals have led women to believe that doctors are in control of their vaginal health. Many women may seek a doctor for issues such as yeast infections or odor; however, manmade chemicals have proven to be unhelpful. Women may have to seek several treatments or continue to use some form of chemical medication. However, natural herbs heal a number of vaginal issues by ridding the vagina of anything preventing the vagina from functioning properly. Unfortunately, there has been an attack on this method of womb healing, especially online via negative or false articles, simply because it actually works!

Although the vagina is self-cleaning, it must be in optimal health in order to do so. If the vagina were in optimal health, women wouldn't experience infertility, odor, or infections. Also, there are certain issues that the vagina cannot cleanse itself of, such as herpes, HPV, and cysts! Women are exposed to chemicals and toxins that cause several vaginal ailments. These pollutants can show themselves through various imbalances, including bacterial vaginosis, yeast infections, endometriosis, infertility, vaginal pain, excess bleeding, vaginal dryness, and fibroids.

Unfortunately, our diets also affect vaginal health more than we know! Consuming large amounts of dairy products like cheese or milk can cause mucus and yeast to build up inside the vagina. Lack of water can cause dryness and itching. Also, medications for other diseases can affect vaginal health. For instance, some diabetic medicine can cause chronic yeast infections in women. There are many factors that contribute to an unhealthy vagina.

As a result, many women suffer from fibroids, cysts, tumors, hot flashes, dryness, and abnormal cervical cells. Also, the toxins from a poor diet, emotional stress, and a chemical-based environment can also affect the vagina. These toxins can cause several imbalances in the vagina, such as bacterial vaginosis, yeast infections, endometriosis, infertility, vaginal pain, excess bleeding or irregular cycles.

Birth control (IUD, the Depo shot, pills) can also affect our bodies negatively. While the goal may be not to conceive, some women use birth control to stop or lighten their cycles. With long-term use, birth control can cause issues with reproducing in the future. Many women have reported odor or BV after having an IUD inserted. Birth control can also have negative effects on hormones as well.

Some women do not have a cycle for weeks, months, or years due to either endometriosis or PCOS. Or, some women may no longer have a cycle to help cleanse their vagina due to a hysterectomy. Therefore, it is important for women to detox their wombs to ensure vaginal health. Other benefits of cleansing with Yummy Yoni Pearls include vaginal tightening, restoration of natural moisture, balanced hormones, and shorter, lighter, less painful cycles.

Many appreciate the benefits of cleansing with Yummy Yoni Pearls. Cycles are not supposed to be painful or more than 3 days long. Cycles are only supposed to last a few minutes to 3 days at the most.

These well-known facts are hidden in negative online press and by the greed of vaginal health care providers. Detoxing is completely safe, if used properly and as directed. The vagina or "yoni" is a temple. The yoni is responsible for the creation of life and must function properly in order to do so or to enjoy life. Yummy Yoni Pearls are produced to help women cleanse, nourish, detoxify, heal, and transform their wombs.

Yummy Yoni Pearls restore the divine feminine energy and the sacredness of the womb by reducing negative energy and negative sexual energy, soul ties, and abuse energies, as well as the elimination of chronic illness and diseases. Womb-detoxing creates the highest energy needed for the conception of a child! Yummy Yoni pearls help clear blockages for a healthier mind, body, and spirit. Yoni pearl is well researched and there is evidence that this natural herb flushes bacteria out of the vaginal canal and cervix.

What is inside Yummy Yoni Pearls?

Yummy Yoni Pearls contain potent, all-natural herbs that help in the removal of toxins from the vagina as it strengthens the uterus, kills parasites and relieves itching. This combination of herbs also helps with hot flashes, pain reduction, and even clearing the mind. The mix of herbal ingredients are absorbed into the body vaginally to expel contents that prevent the vagina from functioning normally. The herbs concentrate on the lower abdomen to help flush and drain the lymphatic system.

Yummy Yoni Pearls' blend of herbs can detox your womb and reset your natural balance, increasing elasticity, regulating the menstrual cycle, killing parasites and bacteria, improving fertility, and reducing discharge. The active ingredients include the following:

1. Motherwort is a traditional herb used for heart conditions, irregular heartbeat or heart symptoms due to anxiety and depression. However, motherwort is also utilized for the absence of menstrual periods, flatulence, and hyperthyroidism or an overactive thyroid. Motherwort also stimulates uterine tone and blood flow, and it reduces menopausal symptoms.

2. Osthol is a type of bicyclic aromatic compound found in many plants. Research shows this substance plays a significant role in liver health and brain function and in the dilation of blood vessels.

3. Angelica is a plant. The seed, root, and fruit of it is used to make medicine. It is used for heartburn, flatulence, loss of appetite, arthritis, circulation problems, nervousness, and insomnia. Angelica can also be used to start menstrual periods. Angelica is useful in increasing urine production, stimulating output and secretion of phlegm, improving sex drive, and killing germs.

4. Borneol has a broad range of uses. Borneol aids the digestive system by stimulating the production of gastric juices. It tones the heart and improves circulation. Borneol can also relieve pain caused by rheumatic diseases, reduce swelling, and

relieve stress. Borneol can be used to promote relaxation and reduce exhaustion.

5. Rhizoma is a root mostly used for stomach weakness and spleen health, diarrhea, and excessive vaginal discharges.

Can I use them?

Any woman born with a vagina who is between the ages of 18 and 65 can use the Yummy Yoni Pearls. If you are pregnant, breastfeeding or a virgin, you cannot detox. If you have an IUD, use one pearl per cleanse. If you have sensitive skin or a sensitive yoni, start with one pearl.

What are the side effects?

Some women may experience the following side effects:

1. Spotting. Yummy Yoni Pearls will regulate your cycle, change cycle patterns, or cause a cycle to start earlier than normal.
2. Light cramps. As the herbs breakdown toxins, some dead vaginal skin cells or tissue may cause slight cramping.
3. Watery discharge. Drinking the recommended amount of water may increase natural moisture as bacteria and toxins are expelled.
4. Itching. As toxins are expelled through the vagina, itching or discomfort is normal. More water will help flush the toxins out quicker, with less itching or irritation.

Are these dangerous?

With proper usage, this detox isn't harmful. Women should only cleanse a maximum of 4 times a month. Several articles have been published on the internet to scare women away from this holistic, ancient healing method; they are instead encouraged to utilize expensive doctors, surgeries, and chemicals. The results pictured can be very shocking as well! These negative articles would say you need this inside of you. However, the content being expelled from your vagina is what is hindering your vagina from functioning properly.

Who developed vaginal detoxing with herbs?

Yummy Yoni Pearls are a form of womb detoxing based on herbalism. Herbalism is a system based on the use of plants or plant extracts to treat diseases, illnesses, etc. Since ancient times, herbal medicine has been used by many different cultures throughout the world to maintain health and for the treatment of illnesses.

The concept of using a combination of herbs for vaginal/reproductive healing and health has been traced back centuries to indigenous China and India and to Native American, African, and Asian cultures. These cultures still use womb detoxing treatment for day-to-day healing purposes. Although, each blend used among the cultures is different, much credit must be given to the traditional Chinese herbs used in our Yummy Yoni Pearls.

Is this FDA approved?

No. However, most herbal treatments aren't. Yummy Yoni Pearls have not been evaluated by the FDA. This product is not intended to diagnose, treat, cure, or prevent disease.

Will this cleanse me of past sexual partners?

The womb detox journey is a spiritual cleanse of the vagina as well. This deeply transformative and healing attunement restores the divine feminine energy within the womb. This sacred detox cleanses the womb of negative or past relationship stress, abuse, and sexual experiences to create the highest energy needed, especially for the conception of a child. Energy exchange is equally as important as a viral, bacterial and physiological exchange between partners occurs. Using the Yummy Yoni Pearls will help in the elimination of blockages for a healthier mind, body and spirit.

When inserting your Yummy Yoni Pearls, recite a positive affirmation or words of intent to energetically detox your womb from the past. See examples below:

"My yoni is a temple. I release the past, I accept my present and only accept positive energy."

"I release negativity and embrace self-love."

"I acknowledge my flaws and free myself of my past to vibe higher in my future."

What can I expect during my detox journey?

Some goddesses experience unreleased or dead vaginal skin cells, old blood clots, yeast, mucus, polyps, scar tissue, and built-up or excessive vaginal tissue from the cervix, uterus, and vaginal walls. Some goddesses experience bleeding due to irregular or heavy cycles. When toxin levels are more than our body's capacity to remove them, buildup occurs.

It's possible to have toxins stored in your body for many years without experiencing any negative symptoms, but the moment the burden of toxins gets too high in your body, you start to feel ill and your fertility declines. Toxins are a hindrance to good health; they trigger your body to release stress hormones into your body.

How do I use them?

Directions: *If you have an IUD or a sensitive Yoni, please use 1 pearl per cleanse.

1. Wash your hands before removing the detox from the sealed package.

2. Unravel the strings and twist three pearls together, from top to bottom.

3. Lay on your back with your knees to your chest.

3. Take the longest finger you have (middle finger) and use it to push the Yummy Yoni Pearls deeply into your vagina. Or remove a super tampon from the plastic and insert pearls. Insert at least 7 cm deep or without discomfort.

4. Leave the 3 Yummy Yoni Pearls in for 3 days or 72 hours.

5. After 72 hours, remove the Yummy Yoni Pearls with clean hands and dispose of them. Squat and gently remove the pearls by pulling the strings.

6. Wear a pantyliner for the next 72 hours, as your vagina will be detoxing.

7. Wait an additional 72 hours to start another cleanse or to have sex.

*If you think you may be sensitive, insert 1 pearl for 24 hours and remove. If no signs of irritation appear, insert remaining 2 pearls for another 48 hours, then remove. Then, continue the detox as directed.

Any tips for a successful detox?

Follow all directions. Drink at least half of your body weight in ounces of water during this process for the best detox results (1 gallon of water for every 100 pounds you weigh). Do not pull detox or toxins, which will come out naturally. Avoid tub baths, sex, and swimming.

What should I NOT do during my detox?

Do NOT cleanse if you think you are pregnant.

Do NOT cleanse while menstruating. Wait 3 days after your cycle ends or 10 before your cycle to conceive.

Do NOT have sexual intercourse while cleansing. Wait 72 hours after your cleanse.

Do NOT reuse.

What if nothing comes out? Did I do it wrong?

If nothing comes out, as far as tissue, that's a good thing! However, bacteria and parasites are also being expelled from the vagina that you can't see. Detoxing isn't all about what comes out; restoring the vagina is the point of the detox. You may not have inserted the pearls deep enough.

What else do I need to know about Yummy Yoni Pearls?

Yummy Yoni Pearls can help treat and prevent various gastrointestinal ailments. In general, women's reproductive organs encounter semen from unprotected sex, birth, miscarriages, abortions, and other blockages or infections that may occur. Yoni pearl is well researched and evidence has proven the blend of natural herbs flush bacteria out of the vaginal canal and cervix. Several women can testify to the natural healing abilities of Yummy Yoni Pearls. Women actively share their stories of healing from cervical cancer to infertility on the official Instagram page of Yummy Yoni Pearls @YummyYoniPearls. More reviews can be found on the official website YummyYoniPearls.net.

Each body has a chakra and an aura that needs and benefits from floral essences that allow the body to vibrate at a healed frequency. These floral waters are produced with herbs, spices, roots, etc. to help our energies vibrate whole and healed for our well-being. The womb and the whole-body aids from this allowing for the mind, body balance and overall healing.

Do you have any success stories?

Yes! Since women are cleansing for different reasons, each woman can experience different results, side effects, etc. However, most women who start cleansing with Yummy Yoni Pearls do not stop. Women love the benefits, effects, and healing they receive from Yummy Yoni Pearls. Here are a few:

Endometriosis is a vaginal disorder that can affect women of any age or race. Endometriosis is usually very painful because tissue that normally lines the inside of your uterus, or the endometrium, is growing outside of the uterus. Endometriosis commonly affects the ovaries, fallopian tubes, and the tissue lining the pelvis. Moreover, the excessive endometrial tissue continues to break down and bleed with each menstrual cycle. Since the vagina is unable to flush this tissue, the buildup becomes trapped inside the vagina, which can cause extreme pain.

This severe pain can worsen during menstruation. Besides the abdominal pains and irregular or heavy cycles, other symptoms may include but are not limited to the following:

Severe cramps

Extended cycles lasting longer than 7 days

Heavy cycles

Painful sex

Infertility

Yummy Yoni Pearls are effective in treating endometriosis because this cleanse will begin to breakdown and remove excessive tissue and lining. It will balance hormones and regulate the cycle to increase fertility. Although 6-7 cleanses are needed for endometriosis, most women suffering from endometriosis notice the difference on their first cleanse. However, with continuous use, women have eliminated pain associated with endometriosis and have even conceived. One goddess informed us her endometriosis decreased significantly, according to her OB/GYN. Also, this goddess is no longer at risk for developing fibrous tissue that can cause pelvic tissues and organs to stick together. Eventually, with continuous cleansing, this goddess will cleanse herself of endometriosis.

Just wanted to give you a new updated. I took my yoni pearls out Aug 17th. Since Sep 1st I've been having big&small blood clots coming out of me. So at first it scared me because I thought "I'm losing a lot of blood" so I made ob/gyn appointment. Come to find out my endometriosis has decreased significantly and no longer at risk of fubriods. @YUMMYYONIPEARLS

Yessss 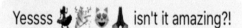 isn't it amazing?!

 Absolutely!!! I'll definitely let you know when my endometriosis is completely gone&&send pics of my future cleanses.

Yesss plz do 😆

YUMMYYONIPEARLS.NET

Just took out your pearls on my first detox. This all came out. I'm going to do it a few more times. And I'll keep you updated but ice recommend it to my cousin who has been having terrible periods.

HH, omg, what were you cleansing for?

I just been noticing a lot of pain during sex recently and that my cycle was really bad. It was 3 pearls, 2.5 days, first cleanse

I also have endometriosis

Ok so please keep me posted and remember you have to keep cleansing. This is wonderful, I'm so happy you got that out of you 😫 HH😼

I know I'm gonna do another. I'll keep you posted thank you

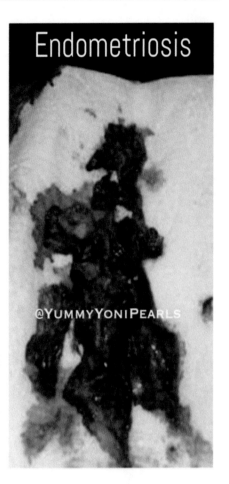

YUMMYYONIPEARLS.NET

Cervical Cancer occurs when abnormal cervical cells reproduce rapidly. Yummy Yoni Pearls have been said to cleanse a number of abnormal cells, such as herpes, HPV, and cancer. One goddess shared that after just 3 Yummy Yoni Pearls cleanses, she was cervical cancer-free!

YummyYoniPearls.net

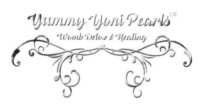

http://YummyYoniPearls.net

Today at 4:47 PM

Im so excited to share 3 months ago 80% of my cervix was covered in cancer cells.

As of today after 3 cleanses 100% CLEAR! @YUMMYYONIPEARLS

Thank u thank you goddess and your products have healed me I feel great God Bless you

YUMMYYONIPEARLS.NET

Heavy or irregular cycles have become a burden for women. Some women experience cycles so painful they cannot get out of bed. Other women experience heavy cycles that last for weeks, even months. Yummy Yoni Pearls are designed to regulate the menstrual cycle, resulting in shorter, lighter, less painful periods! This cleanse will even cause menstruation in women who have not seen a cycle in years.

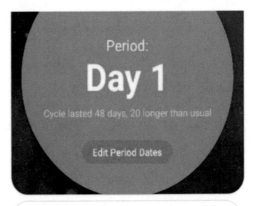

Period:

Day 1

Cycle lasted 48 days, 20 longer than usual

Edit Period Dates

 I think the detox started my cycle

it does regulate your cycle.

 And that's my 2nd detox

Ok cool, are you noticing a difference in your cycles yet?

It's lighter, not heavy at all you're amazing @YUMMYYONIPEARLS

YUMMYYONIPEARLS.NET

Cysts are fluid-filled sacs, which usually come in the form of ovarian cysts or Bartholin cysts.

Ovarian cysts are fluid-filled sacs in the ovaries, commonly formed during ovulation each month. Many women with ovarian cysts don't have symptoms. The cysts are usually harmless. Functional cysts usually go away on their own without treatment; they can be caused by hormonal imbalances or by doctor-prescribed drugs used to help with ovulation. Women with endometriosis can eventually develop endometrioma, which is when endometrial tissue attaches to the ovary and forms a growth. These cysts can be painful during sex and during menstruation. Other symptoms may include bloating, swelling, or pains in the lower abdomen on the side of the cyst, unexplained weight gain, and unusual vaginal bleeding.

Bartholin cysts occur when the Bartholin's glands' ducts are blocked and filled with fluid. The Bartholin's glands are pea-sized glands, found just behind the inner lips that surround the entrance to the vagina known as the labia majora. The purpose of the Bartholin's glands is to secrete fluid, which acts as a lubricant during sex. The fluid travels down tiny tubes and into the vagina. If the ducts become blocked, the buildup of fluid causes the ducts to expand, becoming a cyst. If the cyst or glands become infected, the result can be a painful abscess, which is a collection of growing pus.

Both ovarian and Bartholin cysts are known to return. However, with continuous cleansing with Yummy Yoni Pearls, both types of cysts have been known to reduce in size or disappear completely. The purpose of this cleanse is to expel anything stopping the vagina from functioning properly. Although most cysts do not cause pain or discomfort and aren't cancerous, the risk of ovarian cancer increases with age. Also, any pain with fever and vomiting, sudden and severe abdominal pain, and rapid breathing can be a symptom of a broken open, or ruptured cyst. Larger ruptured cysts can cause heavy bleeding.

Several women have praised Yummy Yoni Pearls after battling with cysts for years. One goddess, who is now a Yummy Yoni Pearls rep, experienced the effects of cleansing for cysts. After 15 years of battling with cysts and fibroids, this goddess was officially cleared of both cysts and fibroids after cleansing! This goddess expressed her joy after receiving the news via phone that she no longer had cysts on her ovaries. For the last few years, this goddess went to the "best" doctors in California for treatment with no results. However, after cleansing, this goddess is getting her womb ready to conceive after years of trying with her husband. Here are a few reviews from other women cleansing for cysts.

@yummyyonipearls so i meant to tell u i have a bartholin cysts and it seemd ro never reduce in size but after this 2nd detox its shrunk dwn quite a bit so im just gonna keep detoxn till it disappear.......OMG im sooo happy about this and u can post this if u want@YummyYoniPearls

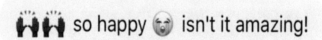 so happy 😭 isn't it amazing!

Yessss

Ok love definitely keep me posted
😆 @YummyYoniPearls

YummyYoniPearls.net

Sure of course told a few coworkers about the yummypearls all us women need this miracle thank you so much

🙌🙌 thank you for sharing!

Today at 12:19 PM

Omg the cyst is gone went to the doctor doctor said nothing is on my ovaries nothing yea some blood came out and tissue I'm so happy

🙌😭 I'm soooo happy for you 🥰 isn't it amazing?!

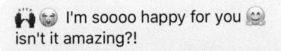

Vaginal abnormalities or blockages are caused by miscarriages, after birth, etc. Here is a review of one woman who had a miscarriage but still had pains. After cleansing with Yummy Yoni Pearls, this goddess passed a blockage, possibly left over from a recent miscarriage.

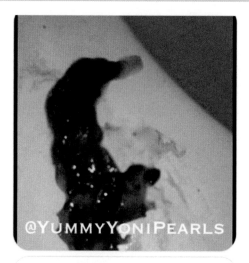

Had a miscarriage a year ago been having a constant pain in my left side ever since. Tried the pearls and this is what came out. Haven't felt that pain anymore. These pearls really work.

Omg 🙌🙌 I'm so happy for you 🥹 this is why I do this 🥰 you just made my day 🤗

YUMMYYONIPEARLS.NET

Where can I purchase Yummy Yoni Pearls?

To start your womb detox journey, visit YummyYoniPearls.net. Also available in stores: 4525 Glenwood Road in Decatur at The Pop Up Shop, and 6525 Tara Blvd in Jonesboro at The Photo Shop.

Can I see more result pics?

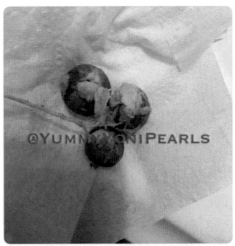

YUMMYYONIPEARLS.NET

 Here is what I discovered after the three days I could see the tissues coming out daily when I showered but this was the final product now my three days of cleanse is going to begin I'm super excited and satisfied thus far!..Thank You!

OMG! I never thought my results would look like this...I'm shocked and ready for my next order. Thanks so much for your advise.

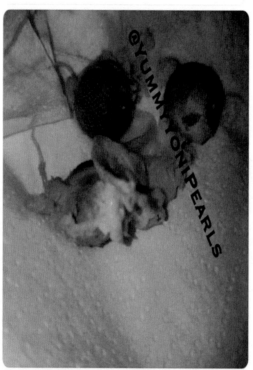

YUMMYYONIPEARLS.NET

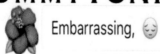 Embarrassing, 😔

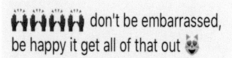 don't be embarrassed, be happy it get all of that out 😺

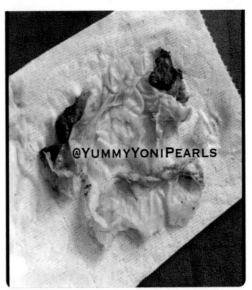

YUMMYYONIPEARLS.NET

I am so shocked and amazed that it
really works like look at all that

Us ladies think that our inside are
clean and look it that

I am satisfied with what I seen and
can't wait to do another detox next
month 🤍

 Thanks Goddess

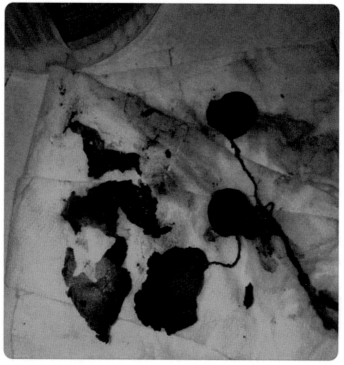

○ Double tap to like

Omg. So I took my pearls out and im embarrassed whats was clogging my uterus. I suffered a miscarriage a couple of months ago. I cant believe this.... This after the 72 hours.

Wow

All the stories, photos, and testimonies in this guide are 100% true and authentic. The women who decided to have faith in Yummy Yoni Pearls have been loyal customers and have become independent distributors of Yummy Yoni Pearls as well.

To learn more about becoming a Yummy Yoni Pearl rep, send an email to **YummyYoniReps@gmail.com**. Our Yummy Yoni Pearls affiliate program is growing with each cleanse sold. Each Yummy Yoni rep has experienced the healing powers of Yummy Yoni Pearls. The goal of the Yummy Yoni Pearls affiliate program is to give every woman, across the globe, an opportunity to share her journey and to sell Yummy Yoni Pearls to other women in need of this detox. Yummy Yoni Pearls are one of the many herbal detoxes sold and manufactured by James & James, LLC.

James & James, LLC, was established by the founder, Jared James, in 2014. Yummy Yoni Pearls is just one of Jared's many profitable online brands, which have started being sold in stores! After his wife and the CEO of James & James, LLC, Mesi James, experienced her first detox, Jared encouraged Mesi to share her story. With more research and the help of distant relatives, Jared and Mesi were ready to create their own brand of yoni pearls. In early 2017, Jared and Mesi launched Yummy Yoni Pearls.

The Jameses have other branches of James & James, LLC, including RAW Passion Photography, Activated Charcoal Tooth Powder, Black Seed Oil, Deep Cleansing Black Facial Mask, and other services/products. The Jameses also give love and business advice in their books, *Young, Black, & Married: How to Snuggle through the Struggle* and *Young, Black, & Married: Teamwork Makes the Dream Work*. To learn more about all the products and services offered by James & James, LLC, visit JamesandJamesLLC.com. To learn more about their book and DVD series, visit YoungBlackandMarried.net.

Follow all the James & James, LLC, brands on Instagram @charcoaltoothpowder, @yummyyonipearls, @wearethejames, @_thepopupshop, and @_thephotoshop_. The goal of James & James, LLC, is to rebuild Black Wall Street, one brick at a time, starting with the family!

Made in the USA
Coppell, TX
13 May 2022

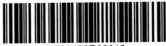

77725483R00019